Explore the Mysterious Link
Between Your Life and Your Body

15 Fascinating Things That Demonstrate the Connection Between Your Life-Issues and Body Pain or Illness

There is a relationship between your life-issues and physical pain in, or injury to, certain body parts. If, for example, you are experiencing pain in your lower back, you may be undergoing money problems. Pain in your shoulders may indicate stress from the way you carry your burdens. This Itty Bitty® book is filled with affirmations that address the problems associated with body pain and life-issues.

The difficulties can be approached from the body parts themselves or by visiting www.ittybittypublishing.com and pulling a body part card. Discover the issue and get your affirmation for the day.

Body part issues can include:

- Elbows, which involve establishing boundaries.
- Pelvis, which involves creativity.
- Buttocks, which are your seat of power.

If learning how Body-Life issues are connected interests you, pick up a copy of this remarkable Itty Bitty® book today.

Your Amazing
Itty Bitty®
Body-Life
Connection Book

15 Simple Steps to Understanding
The Connection
Between Your Body and Your Life-Issues

To be used on-line with Body-Life Cards

http://www.ittybittypublishing.com/78212/Body-Wisdom-Cards.htm

Select "Card Reading Tab"

Suzy Prudden &
Joan Meijer-Hirschland

Published by Itty Bitty® Publishing
A subsidiary of S & P Productions, Inc.

Printed in the United States of America

Itty Bitty® Publishing
311 Main Street, Suite D
El Segundo, CA 90245
(310) 640-8885

ISBN: 978-0-9987597-5-3

We would like to dedicate this book to all our Itty Bitty authors who are working so hard and given so much! They have taken the risk of becoming authors and businessmen and women. They inspire us to be bigger and better and to learn more every day.

Stop by our Itty Bitty® website to get your daily Itty Bitty® Body-Life Connection Readings. If you have pain or illness in any body part, have difficulty with body part issues, or draw the body part card on www.ittybittypublishing.com, include affirmations for this body part in your daily life.

http://www.ittybittypublishing.com/78212/Body-Wisdom-Cards.htm

To find out about our Create Your Body-Life New Year Workshop, visit us at:

www.ittybittypublishing.com

Spend the day with Suzy and Joan creating your coming year using the power of your mind.

Table of Contents

Introduction

Your body and your mind are directly connected to major issues in your life. Pain or illness in a part of the body reflects what is happening in your life.

To work with Body-Life Issues, notice where pain or illness is affecting your body. Ask your *Higher Self* what you need to know about the way you are treating yourself and the way others are treating you at this time.

When you have an answer, ask your *Higher Self* what you need to do to change the areas of your life that you don't like. Write your question with your dominant hand (the one you normally write with), receive the answers with your non-dominant hand.

Do not judge any answers you receive. Do not get in your own way with doubts about your ability to do whatever comes to your mind. Simply write down what comes to you. Find the affirmation that you feel best suits your needs in this moment, or make up your own affirmation, one that you feel more closely satisfies your needs. Write the affirmation on a 3 x 5 card. Ask for what you want and expect things to change.

Carry your card with you, rather than posting it somewhere where you will soon forget about it. Read it numerous times during the day. (If you post it, it will soon become invisible to you and you will get no benefit from it.)

In this Itty Bitty® book we precede all affirmations with the words "It's now okay...." The use of "It's now okay" avoids an internal argument between you and your mind if you say something you don't yet believe. For example if you were to say "I am now a millionaire" and you were not a millionaire, your mind would argue. But if you say "It's now okay for me to be a millionaire," the mind would accept that concept. Without the "It's now okay..." your affirmation might not work in a positive way, particularly when you are dealing with major issues.

In this book we are dealing with major body parts. If you want more specific body parts and many more affirmations, order our "Body-Life Connection Book" online.

Body Part 1
Head, Brain and Nerves

Your head or skull represents your *Self* in the world. Your skull is the protective covering that houses your brain/mind — that part of *you* that allows you to function as a living being. You could say your skull symbolizes your *Self-*Protection. The brain, which is housed inside your skull, monitors the needs of every single cell every single minute of your life.

1. Your mind holds your beliefs and thoughts. It produces what's termed "monkey mind," as well as the still small voice of intuition.
2. Your head and mind involve issues of trust and beliefs in yourself.
3. Brain and head injuries are the outward manifestation of victimization and powerlessness. In some cases, brain injuries result in the actual loss of *Self*.
4. Your nerves communicate with every body part. If you have nerve pain, numbness or cannot feel in a certain area of your body, look up the body part to assess the more exact issues you are dealing with.

Affirmations for Your Head and Brain

Head
- It's now okay to trust myself.
- It's now okay to know I am safe.
- It's now okay to trust that my outcomes are perfect in present time.

Brain
- It's now okay to recognize the difference between monkey mind and intuition.
- It's now okay to trust my intuition.
- It's now okay to move in the world without fear or judgment.
- It's now okay to be myself.

Nerves
- It's now okay to communicate with every part of my body.
- It's now okay to receive information about illness and injury. (Draw a second card to specify body part for issue.)
- It's now okay to receive information about my life.

Body Part 2
Face:
Eyes, Ears, Nose and Mouth

Your face is the mirror of your soul. It represents what you show the world. It also symbolizes what you hide from yourself and the world.

1. Your eyes represent what you see in the world, what you see in your life and your attitude toward what you see.
2. Your ears represent your capacity and willingness to hear and to take in and assimilate information. They also tell you whether you are comfortable with your surroundings, or with what other people or situations in your life are "telling" you.
3. Your nose represents self-recognition, awareness of yourself in the world and how comfortable you are with that understanding. It also indicates whether or not you want to be noticed or if you prefer to be invisible.
4. Your mouth is the gateway for both nourishment and expression. It represents taking in new thoughts and ideas and breaking them down into useful form.

Affirmations for Your Face, Eyes, Ears, Nose and Mouth.

Face
- It's now okay to know who I am.
- It's safe to show the world who I am.

Eyes
- It's now okay to see what I need to see.
- It's now okay to envision the perfection of my life and the world around me.

Ears
- It's now okay to hear what is spoken and unspoken.
- It's now okay to listen without judgment or fear.

Nose
- It's now okay to know I'm perfect just the way I am.
- It's now okay to love and approve of myself.

Mouth
- It's now okay to know what I need to say at all times and to express myself easily and effortlessly.
- It's now okay to be able to break down ideas into usable forms that nourish and support me.

Body Part 3
Neck and Shoulders

Your neck represents balance, flexibility and how you perceive and hold life. It serves as the conduit for information between the mind and the body. It represents the ability to perceive what surrounds you, what you just left, what you are going through and where you are going. Shoulders represent the way you carry responsibility. They also represent how you support yourself and those around you.

1. When you have pain or stiffness in your neck, you are being asked to look at where you are out of balance or inflexible in your life.
2. What do you perceive about yourself and others around you?
3. When you have pain or stiffness in your shoulders, you are being asked to look at how you carry responsibility.
4. Do you allow your responsibilities to weigh you down?
5. How do you support yourself and others emotionally, psychologically, spiritually and physically?

Affirmations for Your Neck and Shoulders

Neck

- It's now okay be flexible and to live in balance.
- It's now okay to know that I am safe and to be peaceful in my life.
- It's now okay to be honest with myself.
- It's now okay to be perceived as I really am.
- It's now okay to see all sides of a situation.

Shoulders

- It's now okay to carry my burdens lightly.
- It's now okay to let go of what's weighing me down.
- It's now okay to experience my responsibilities with ease.
- It's now okay to accept responsibility.
- It's now okay to experience my life with ease.

Body Part 4
Throat

The throat represents the channel of expression. It is also the passage for creativity and the pathway through which ideas travel toward the process of digestion and assimilation. It is the route through which life-giving air reaches the lungs and food and water reach the stomach and is therefore a passageway of life sustenance.

1. Problems with the throat, particularly a sore throat, often indicate that you are not saying what you need or want to say in a given circumstance.
2. Problems in swallowing may indicate that you are having difficulty taking in new thoughts and ideas.
3. A "lump in your throat" indicates overwhelming unexpressed emotion, generally sadness.
4. When you have throat issues, you are asked to look at what you are saying and not saying in a given circumstance.
5. You are also being asked to look at how you are taking in and assimilating creative ideas and suggestions.

Affirmations for the Throat

Affirmations for the throat include what you say and what you don't say.

Throat

- It's now okay to express myself, even the things I am reluctant to say.
- It's now okay to accept in my life, the things that interest me and the things that empower me.
- It's now okay to express my emotions.
- It's now okay to trust my voice.
- It's now okay to know it's safe to say what I need to say.

Body Part 5
Upper Arms and Elbows

It is astonishing how different upper arms and elbows are in terms of the way they play out in life. Upper arms encircle and embrace everything life has to offer. Elbows are sharp, pushing through, elbowing out of the way. The symbolism of elbows involves establishing boundaries. Issues involve invasion of your boundaries.

1. Upper arms represent the joy or discouragement you feel with everything you experience. If you are encountering pain, weight gain or weakness in your upper arms, you may be holding yourself back from experiencing life's adventures fully and completely.

2. Do you have difficulty maintaining boundaries? Are other people constantly violating your boundaries? Are you constantly violating the boundaries of others? Are you constantly "Elbowing in?" Elbows are also a symbol of aggression. "Elbowing your way" through a crowd is part of the English lexicon, as is "Making elbow room."

Affirmations for Upper Arms and Elbows and Upper Arm and Elbow Issues

Upper Arms
- It's now okay to embrace life fully, with joy and ease
- It's now okay to know it's okay to fully experience my life.
- It's now okay to know all aspects of my life are perfect in every way.
- It's now okay to move forward and enjoy my life experiences.
- It's now okay to know life is my experience.

Elbows
- It's now okay to establish and maintain my boundaries easily and effortlessly.
- It's now okay to express my boundary needs and requirements.
- It's now okay to relinquish my need to violate the boundaries of others.
- It's now okay to be at ease with asking for my space.
- It's now okay to respect my own boundaries and the boundaries of others.

Body Part 6
Lower Arms, Wrist, Hands and Fingers

It is astonishing how different these adjoining body parts are.

1. Lower arms represent balancing what you carry in life. Or a tendency to juggle many things at once. Lower arms represent your willingness or resistance to reaching out and asking for assistance.

2. Your wrists represent your ability to move with ease while handling all aspects of your life. They also represent how you move in your life: fluidly, rigidly, lightly, with ease or with difficulty. Your wrists symbolize how you accept or reject pleasure in your life.

3. Your hands represent the ability to grasp and manage life. They also represent the limitations you put on yourself, your skillfulness and dexterity at managing things.

4. Your fingers represent the details of your life. There is an implication of deftness, physical skill, dexterity when it comes to the fingers. Fingers focus more on managing the little things with adroit strength. Fingers also express nervousness, boredom and pent up energy.

Affirmations for Lower Arms, Wrists, Hands and Fingers

Lower Arms

- It's now okay to balance all aspects of my life easily and effortlessly.
- It's now okay to celebrate my experiences and welcome assistance as I juggle my life.

Wrists

- It's now okay to manage all my experiences with wisdom and love with ease.
- It's now okay to move through life easily and effortlessly.

Hands

- It's now okay to handle all aspects of my life with joy and ease.
- It's now okay to experience and express my emotions safely.

Fingers

- It's now okay to enjoy taking care of the details of my life.
- It's now okay to recognize that trivia isn't necessarily trivial.

Step 7
Chest and Breasts

Chest and breasts may appear to be the same thing and they definitely complement each other, but they are not the same.

1. Your chest represents the ability to give and take in love and life safely. Pain in the chest, depending on where it is located, can be associated with fear, guilt, anger, repression, rigidity and grief. The chest is also the center of giving. When the ability to give or receive is blocked, pain in the chest (heart or lungs) may follow.
2. Your breasts represent nurturing and nourishing yourself and others. They also represent nourishment, both physically, as in food, and emotionally – as in feelings. When one does not get enough nourishment, either from others or from oneself, one may experience breast discomfort. When a woman is a nurturer, but does not enjoy being a nurturer, or finds herself giving to others at her own expense, she may experience breast problems. Breasts also represent a woman's feeling about her own femininity and sensuality.

Affirmations for the Breasts and Chest

Breasts

- It's now okay to be balanced in giving and receiving love and care.
- It's now okay to allow myself to be nurtured.
- It's now okay to give without depleting myself.
- It's now okay to ask for and receive what I need.
- It's now okay to receive as much as I give.

Chest

- It's now okay to take in and utilize all of life's loving experiences.
- It's now okay to love my life exactly as it is.
- It's now okay to ask for what I want and receive it.
- It's now okay to love without expectations.
- It's now okay to make the changes I want in my life successfully, easily, effortlessly and lovingly.
- It's now okay to love and give to myself.

Body Part 8
Heart and Lungs

The respiratory and circulatory systems are team players. Under the direction of the mind, the lungs work hand-in-hand with the heart and circulatory system to sustain your body and your life.

1. The heart represents the center of love and empowerment. It is the energy force for moving your life in any direction you want to go. The heart is powerful, it is not logical. The heart and the mind work as a team. Without each other, the heart and the mind are incomplete halves. The heart contains your passion, your joy, your lust for life. Your mind directs the power of your heart.
2. Breathing is synonymous with life. Your lungs represent your ability to fully take in life. It is also synonymous with ridding life and your body of physical, mental and emotional toxins. Your respiratory system is the Yin to your circulatory system's Yang. Diseases of the lung generally interfere with your respiratory system's ability to bring in life-sustaining oxygen or eliminate toxic carbon dioxide.

Affirmations for the Heart and Lungs

Heart

- It's now okay to love and be loved.
- It is now okay for my heart energy to move me in any direction I want to go.
- It is now okay to realize my passion.
- It is now okay to celebrate the joy of living.
- It is now okay to rejoice in my lust for life.

Lungs

- It's now okay to trust and feel safe in my life.
- It is now okay for me to enjoy the breath of life.
- It is now okay for me to work as part of an effective team.
- It is now okay for me to eliminate the toxic elements in my life easily and effortlessly.
- It is now okay for me to enjoy my powerful life force.

Step 9
Upper, Midriff, Lower Back, Stomach

This entire area of the body deals with heightened emotions, safety and security in various forms.

1. The upper back represents safety, support, love and trust. Pain in the upper back can often mean fear, either of giving or receiving love or not being able to trust either oneself or someone else.
2. Your midriff represents how you deal with your emotions, with ease or difficulty, with confidence or fear. Your midriff stores or embraces your emotions. Weight around the midriff may indicate a need for extra protection in the area of emotions.
3. The lower back represents support. Pain in the lower back occurs when there is a deep subconscious fear that there is "not enough." In many cases, the fear revolves around money. Lower back problems may mean a lack of trust that there will always be enough in life. Fear and trust cannot exist in the same space.
4. Your abdomen houses your creativity and gut reactions. Stomach problems may indicate a blockage in your life. You may be feeling trapped, or stuck.

Affirmations for Your Upper Back, Midriff, Lower Back and Stomach

Upper Back

- It's now okay to receive love, guidance and support from known and unknown sources.
- It's now okay to know that life and God support me.

Midriff

- It's now okay to trust that all negative emotions will pass with time.
- It's now okay to stop blaming others for my emotions.

Lower Back

- It's now okay to know that all my needs are met in present time.
- It's now okay to receive money from expected and unexpected sources.

Stomach (Abdomen)

- It's now okay to fully digest all that comes to me.
- It is now okay for me to follow my inner knowing.

Step 10
Hips and Pelvis

Your hips and pelvis deal with imbalance and not moving forward in your life. Whether you are dealing with creativity or an imbalance between work and play, hips suggest a need for change.

1. Your hips represent balance and forward motion. If you have problems in your hips, your life may be out of balance or you may be overloaded in one area (work versus play). It may also mean you are holding yourself back. If you have pain in your hips, you may want to look at where you are not moving forward. If you are out of balance or stuck in your life, in your job or in your relationships, your hips will tell the tale.
2. Your pelvis holds creativity and sexuality; the expression of your life force. When there is pain in the pelvic area or discomfort you may be experiencing a holding back or blockage of your creativity. You may be living life less fully than you really want to be living. You may be in a situation you don't know how to get out of, or doing that which you don't want to do.

Affirmations for Your Hip and Pelvis Issues

Hips

- It's now okay to have balance in my life and move myself forward with ease.
- It's now okay to know I am free to move forward in my life in perfect balance.
- It's now okay to play.
- It's now okay to rest and take care of myself.
- It's now okay to move on from that which does not serve me.

Pelvis

- It's now okay to express the life force that lives within me.
- It's now okay to fully express my creativity.
- It's now okay to live the life I want to live.
- It's now okay to enjoy my sexuality.
- It's now okay to fully express my creativity.

Step 11
Buttocks

Your buttocks are all about power. Whether you are threatened by someone else's power or you cannot express your own power, your buttocks will let you know.

1. Your buttocks are your seat of power. When you have excess weight on the buttocks, it usually means fear of your own power or an inability to access or express your power.
2. The buttocks hold the power that you are afraid of, or are unwilling or unable to express.
3. When the buttocks are out of shape, power is mishandled, loosely held or blocked.

It is particularly interesting that in this culture, large buttocks are more of a female problem than a male problem.

Affirmations for your Buttocks

Buttocks

- It's now okay to know I am safe in my power and the power of others.
- It's now okay to trust and be comfortable with my power.
- It's now okay to own my power.
- It's now okay to know that my power attracts power.
- It's now okay to know that, if power is being abused, I can leave.
- It's now okay to know I'm okay.

Step 12
Thighs and Knees

Thighs and knees, when positive, represent forward motion and flexibility. When pain or injury affect these areas look for fear, weakness, inflexibility and anger.

1. Thighs represent strength and forward motion. They hold repressed anger and past powerlessness. Excess weight on the thighs may mean you are holding on to the past or negative childhood memories associated with anger and rage. You may experience pain in or injury to your thighs if you are unable to express the anger, you are constantly afraid or feel powerless to act on your own behalf.
2. Knees represent flexibility, inflexibility, pride and ego. Pain in or injury to the knee may mean there is lack of flexibility in your life.

Affirmations for Your Thighs and Knees

Thighs
- It's now okay to release the past, heal my rage and move forward with ease.
- It's now okay to forgive all childhood trespasses, real and imagined, and go forth to positive feelings.
- It's now okay to love life and enjoy my present experiences.
- It's now okay to express my anger and release it.
- It's now okay to move beyond the past and enjoy the present.

Knees
- It's now okay to have a working relationship with my ego and my pride.
- It's now okay to love my ego and partner with it to make my life work.
- It's now okay to be flexible in every aspect of my life.
- It's now okay to bend and flow with ease.
- It's now okay to have balanced pride.

Step 13
Calves, Ankles, Feet and Toes

Here is the area of your base, forward motion, foundation and stability. If you have life-issues in these areas, it is time to look at where you are stuck and where you have released your strength.

1. Your lower legs carry you forward in life. When there is pain or injury, you may be stopping yourself. When there is extra weight, you may feel the need to weigh yourself down, to slow yourself in your forward movement.
2. Your ankles represent the way you move through and deal with change.
3. Your feet are the base upon which you stand. They are the foundation that supports you even as you move forward in your life, take action and reach for your dreams.
4. Your toes represent the minor details of the future each in slightly different ways. They include: your personal will, whether you follow through with all the minor details of your life, your ambition, your leadership ability and your willingness to follow your intention.

Affirmations for Calves, Ankles, Feet & Toes and the Life-Issues Associated With Them.

Calves

- It's now okay for me to move myself forward in my life safely and with ease.
- It's now okay to step out into the world.

Ankles

- It's now okay to change direction easily and effortlessly.
- It's now okay to move in any direction with ease and flexibility.

Feet

- It's now okay to create a strong foundation in my life.
- It's now okay to move forward with strength and security.

Toes

- It's now okay to be present and aware as I set up my future.
- It's now okay to pay attention and move with confidence and security.

Step 14
Muscles and Bones

Bones form the structure that muscles hold together in both your body and your life. Bone and muscle issues have severe impacts on other parts of the body.

1. Your muscles hold the whole structure of your body and life together. They allow you to hold yourself together. They let you move. When muscles are sore, it may mean you are having difficulty moving within the structure of your life. It may be too structured, or you may not have enough structure. Weakness may indicate you do not have the strength to move your life in the direction you want. Inflexibility may be a sign of holding yourself back.

2. Your bones represent structure. When you have bone problems, you may feel rebellious against the structure of society, your home life, or the way you have structured your life. You may have a strong "Don't tell me what to do" vibe, compensating for a feeling of weakness in the face of adversity or the rule of the society you live in. Injury may give you time to contemplate your needs.

Affirmations for Muscles and Bones

Muscles

- It's now okay to move easily within the structure of my life.
- It's now okay to allow myself the freedom to move with ease in any direction.
- It's now okay to balance all areas of my life.
- It's now okay to be strong in my life.
- It's now okay to hold myself together as I move forward in my life.

Bones

- It's now okay to get out of my own way.
- It's now okay to move in the direction I want to go.
- It's now okay to stop when I need to.
- It's now okay to choose a new tribe.
- It's now okay to recognize discipline is freedom.

Step 15
Skin

Your skin is the largest organ in your body. It makes you waterproof. It is one of the organs that allows you to be in touch with the world around you. It protects you from deadly germs and infections.

1. Your skin senses and protects. It guards your individuality. Problems with your skin show a lack of belief in your own individuality. It may indicate you feel invaded by others.
2. Your skin is a sensory organ. When you have skin problems, you may be denying your senses, not allowing yourself to fully hear, see, feel, taste or smell.
3. Sensing also means allowing yourself to intuit situations. Skin problems may be the manifestation of your inability or unwillingness to follow your own sense of knowing.

Affirmations for Your Skin

Skin

- It's now okay to pay attention to my senses as they guide and protect me in the world.
- It's now okay to know I am safe being me.
- It's now okay to trust my sense of knowing.
- It's now okay to know I am safe in the world.
- It's now okay to enjoy the richness of my life.

You've finished. Before you go...

Tweet/share that you finished this book.

Please star rate this book.

Reviews are solid gold to writers. Please take a few minutes to give us some itty bitty feedback.

ABOUT THE AUTHORS

SUZY PRUDDEN made her stage debut in a dance recital at the age of two as the lead elephant in a long line of two-year olds in a rendition of "The Circus." It was love at first performance. Suzy never again saw a stage she didn't want to be on – preferably in the center.

As a successful entrepreneur, she founded Suzy Prudden Studios – the first, largest and most successful toddler exercise school in New York City, a business that propelled her to 13 books, twenty national tours, The Today Show, Good Morning America and Oprah, along with hundreds of magazines and newspapers. After selling her fitness company she opened a hypnosis center working with weight loss. She added entrepreneurs to her client base in the early 2000s. She next started coaching her business hypnosis clients in how to grow their companies. On the way, she and her sister Joan Meijer-Hirschland wrote "The Itty Bitty Weight Loss Book" and discovered a unique blend of publishing and business building.

Together they formed the Itty Bitty® Publishing Community which publishes Itty Bitty® Books – 15 Simple Informative Steps by Experts in Fields of All Kinds and matches them with opportunities for marketing that helps their writers grow their businesses, as well as sell their books.

JOAN MEIJER-HIRSCHLAND has been co-author for Suzy Prudden's last five books. They have discovered that the only way they can work effectively together is on the phone and more recently, Skype, as they've found that working in the same room is hopelessly distracting. Several years ago, at the age of 70, Meijer discovered that she could write erotic short stories – and often drolly recounts how audiences sit up in their chairs at seminars and lean forward when she rolls onto a stage in her wheelchair and informs them she writes erotica under the a pen name – Joan Russell.

She also writes medical thrillers under the pen name John Russell; alternative histories and non-fiction under Joan Meijer; and books about writing, plus the Itty Bitty® Books series under Joan Meijer-Hirschland.

Don't forget to get your Body-Life Connection Readings at:

www.ittybittypublishing.com
Select Card Reading Tab

If you enjoyed this Itty Bitty® Book, you might also enjoy…

- **Your Amazing Itty Bitty® Heal Your Body Book** – Patricia Garza Pinto

- **Your Amazing Itty Bitty® Astrology Book** – Carol Pilkington

- **Your Amazing Itty Bitty® Affirmations Book** – Micaela Pissari

…or the many other Itty Bitty® Books available online

Made in the USA
Middletown, DE
30 June 2022